SUGAR DETOX DIET RECIPES FOR KIDS

A Complete and Healthy Treat for Children

Mclan O. Micheals, RDN.

Disclaimer

The information in this book is intended solely for informational and educational purposes. This book is not intended to provide medical advice and should not be used to diagnose or treat any medical issue. This is a general healthy eating plan, it does not guarantee weight loss and may not be appropriate for everyone depending on certain health conditions & goals. Always consult with a healthcare provider before starting any diet.

Copyright © 2023 Mclan O. Micheals, RDN.

All rights reserved.

Table of Contents

Introduction

Every night while I was growing up, our family had dessert. Usually, it was ice cream. I never ate lunch without a Twinkie or Suzie-Q. It was difficult for me to give up the similar sweet treat traditions with my own family when I became a parent. I felt bad because my kids weren't receiving the same things I did when I was a youngster. It took me a while to recognize that my childhood custom had developed into an adult sugar habit. I was aware that I didn't want to impart it to my kids.

Like my family, most families make an effort to maintain a healthy lifestyle by participating in sports and exercise, cooking at home, and making wise food choices. Sometimes we may be giving our family more added sugar than we plan to without even recognizing it. In recent years, sugar detoxification, sometimes known as "sugar detox," has developed into a method for learning about the added sugar in foods and for changing one's diet and lifestyle.

This book is intended to provide parents with the knowledge and resources they need to assist their kids in living healthy and happy life by limiting their sugar consumption. All parents want their kids to grow up healthy, content, and successful, but it may be challenging to make sure they're eating a balanced diet due to the abundance of sugary foods and beverages in modern culture.

Studies have shown that consuming too much sugar may result in several health issues, including obesity, type 2 diabetes, and heart disease. As a result, there is rising worry about how much sugar youngsters consume. The Sugar Detox Diet for Kids offers a framework for parents to assist their children in reducing their sugar consumption while still allowing them to enjoy scrumptious and healthy meals. It is an effective strategy to address these difficulties.

This book emphasizes achieving a balance and forming lifelong healthy habits rather than depriving children of the pleasures of childhood indulgences. We will look at how sugar affects kids' health, the advantages of a sugar detox diet for kids, and doable strategies to live a low-sugar lifestyle. Parents may assist their kids in maintaining a healthy, balanced diet and putting them on the road to lifelong health with the correct resources and techniques.

Therefore, this book offers everything you need to get started on the road to a better, low-sugar lifestyle for your children, whether you're a concerned parent hoping to enhance your child's health or a caregiver seeking to improve the diet of the children in your care. Let's dig in and begin learning about the Sugar Detox Diet for the Kids' world!

Chapter One

Introduction to Sugar Detox Diet for Kids

Refined sugar is a common food nowadays, and it may be found in bread, cereal, juice, muesli bars, and cookies. While the majority of us are aware that too much sugar is hazardous for our children, it can be quite easy to take more than is advised, which is one reason why they need a detox.

What is Sugar Detox?

When you decide to eliminate as much sugar as you can from your diet for a certain period, you are engaging in a sugar detox.

Why Is Kids' Sugar Detox Important?

For the sake of your child's health, additional sugars must be eliminated from their diet or greatly reduced. It's crucial to instill in your kid proper eating practices. As kids start to exercise freedom and autonomy in their decisions, this will improve the likelihood that they will continue to have a balanced lifestyle.

Taking Steps to Lower the Risk of Health Complications

The preservation of your child's health is the main advantage of cutting down on or eliminating sugar from their diet. The greatest method to lower your child's chance of developing diseases that may have serious and long-lasting effects on their health is to closely monitor added sugar intake.

Establishing the Bases for a Healthy Adulthood

This will pass for a typical meal if your child is used to consuming highly processed or sweetened foods. They won't recognize that these meals don't provide enough nourishment. They are more inclined to stay with what they are familiar with when they make their own dietary decisions.

If you normalize entire foods and balanced meals, your youngster will start to associate healthier food options with eating. When they're adolescents and sometimes have to cook for themselves, they'll be more inclined to make a straightforward, wholesome meal. When sweet cereal isn't something they often eat, they'll desire scrambled eggs with greens instead.

How to Begin the Diet for Sugar Detoxification

Sugar cannot be eliminated from a child's diet. You can't educate your children on how to make wise decisions if you never let them indulge in treats like birthday cake or a snow cone at the beach. Helping children develop their ability to make balanced decisions is increasingly crucial.

Your children won't always be children. They'll be in their late teens and off to college in the space of a single blink. You want them to be able to properly feed themselves when that time comes. They'll be less inclined to stock up on ice cream if they relate it to a good day out with their family.

They'll relate it to a humorous experience or a noteworthy event. You should treat additional sugars in that manner.

Your regular meals and the easy-to-grab snacks you keep around the home shouldn't include a lot of added sugar. Juice drinks and other items often include a lot of added sugar. A better option is to replace them with flavored seltzers. Pick healthy snacks like low-fat yogurt, popcorn, whole fruits, and turkey jerky.

It's as easy as choosing healthy foods to put on the table for your kids when you make meals. You may reduce the amount of sugar in your meals by using whole foods when you cook and avoiding processed or pre-packaged sauces.

For busy parents, making wholesome meals may be challenging. For parents who only have time to prepare complex meals once or twice a week, cooking meals in large quantities ahead of time may be a practical answer.

The key is to have easy, fast, and nutritious options available. Purchasing frozen steam-in-bag veggies and a prepared rotisserie chicken from the deli at your neighborhood grocery shop is quite OK. It simply takes a few minutes to throw together a healthy lunch.

There are grilled selections and side salads at several drive-through restaurants. When things become hectic, keep these things in mind.

Chapter Two

Understanding the Effects of Sugar on Kids

When you take the following into account, you can understand why sugar is such a hard addiction to break:

- Cocaine is 8 times less addictive than sugar.

- Every year, the typical American eats more than 50 pounds of hidden sugar.

- We may believe that we are avoiding sugar, but the fact is that we have no clue how many foods we consume including hidden sugars. Because almost everything we buy at the grocery store, from spaghetti sauce to plain yogurt, has some refined sugar, it becomes increasingly difficult to limit our children's sugar consumption.

Take a look at the effects of sugar on our children:

The Immune System of Your Child Is Suppressed

Sugar might weaken your child's immune system and reduce their ability to fight off infectious diseases. This implies that your kid may be vulnerable to various diseases, such as the flu and other common colds.

Suggestion

All of us want our children to grow up healthy and happy, therefore limiting their sugar consumption. Fruit like blueberries (which strengthens the brain), bananas (which reduces stress), or raw honey on a piece of bread should take the place of those sweet snacks. Remember that while honey contains sugar, it is a genuine food and is a rich source of nutrients that support the immune system.

Sugar Lowers Concentration Levels and Makes Children More Hyperactive

Sugar may cause a child's adrenaline levels to spike quickly, which can make them hyperactive, anxious, unable to focus, and generally cranky.

Suggestion

What foods should I feed my children for breakfast and what do I pack in their lunchboxes? Throw out the sugary cereals and quick meals at lunchtime. Give your kids an egg for breakfast since choline improves brain function. Bring a banana with them for lunch; the potassium in them helps kids focus and remain awake all day.

Sugar Impairs Vision

The amount of sugar your children eat can affect their blood sugar levels and cause the lens of their eyes to enlarge, which will affect how well they can see. Their vision may return to normal if your child is off sugar, or at least not ingesting large quantities of sugar.

Suggestion

Eliminate the sugar from your child's diet and encourage them to consume lutein and zeaxanthin-rich foods like broccoli, avocados, eggs, and carrots if you want them to have good vision. Oils like cod liver oil are excellent for enhancing vision. And no, the lemon-flavored cod liver oil is not unpleasant to taste.

Sugar May Result in Indigestion, Stomach Discomfort, and an Acidic Digestive Tract

Do your kids often experience stomach pain? Indigestion or acid reflux? Do they often consume sugar-containing meals like sodas, candies, or cookies?

In addition to indigestion, an acidic digestive system, and poor vitamin and mineral absorption, sugar consumption may result in several gastrointestinal issues. This may affect how your children feel about school and their capacity to grasp, learn, and take in knowledge.

Suggestion

Bananas, brown rice, sweet potatoes, yogurt, or oatmeal are all good soothing stomach foods to add to your child's diet if they have regular stomach aches or indigestion.

Increased Asthma in Children and Adolescents Is Linked to Sugar

Researchers have discovered a connection between sugar consumption and the rise in asthma cases among children and teenagers. Sonja Kiertein, Ph.D., of the Nestle Research Center in Switzerland, discovered that a high-sugar diet triggers allergic inflammation in the airways' immune system. Inflammation may lead to airway constriction, mucus production, and asthma symptoms such as wheezing and shortness of breath.

Suggestion

Per Adventure your kid has asthma, look at their diet to determine whether sugar is the cause. If that's the case, swap out the sugary treats with fruit instead, such as blueberries, strawberries, or kiwis.

Diabetes Can Be Caused by Sugar in Young People

When children consume excessive amounts of sugar, their insulin sensitivity may decline, leading to unusually high insulin levels and ultimately diabetes. According to research, diabetes is becoming more common among American youth under the age of 20. Their blood vessels, kidneys, nerves, and eyes may all be seriously harmed by this terrible illness. One of the most crippling adverse consequences of sugar on young individuals is this.

Suggestion

Do you consume soda as parents? consume sweet snacks? Eat the majority of your meals at fast food and dining establishments. Or do you prepare your meals at home with your children and consume plenty of wholesome grains, fruits, and vegetables as well as water? Do your kids see you choose healthy snacks like almonds, plain yogurt, or cheese instead of sweet ones? Teach your children how to be healthy and happy. Be their mentor and role model.

Sugar May Be Linked to Children's Food Allergies

Numerous kids and adults struggle with allergies brought on by a variety of causes.

Anaphylaxis, a severe allergic response that may be lethal, can result from an allergy that is strong enough to be combined with meals that include sugar. Children may indeed develop sugar allergies.

Suggestion

Although a scenario of this kind is probably uncommon, it is something to be aware of. Make sure you are keeping a close eye on your child's food if they are prone to allergies. Make it as devoid of sugar as you can.

Children's Eczema May Be Linked to Sugar

Eczema is an inflammatory skin disorder that may affect younger or older children. Doctors advise parents to monitor their child's consumption of sugary foods, such as processed meals and fast food, since they might promote flare-ups of eczema. Why? because sugar raises insulin levels, which leads to inflammation.

Just a little note: When our daughter was a year old, she once had eczema. She was eating a balanced diet with minimal added sugar. My nutrition lessons revealed that low vitamin A levels are a common cause of eczema in kids. We were advised by our pediatric dermatologist to give her 1 teaspoon of lemon-flavored cod liver oil per day, and add 1 tablespoon of raw apple cider vinegar daily, said our. The mixture was effective and the eczema is gone!

Suggestion

Remove as much sugar from your child's diet as you can if they have eczema. Additionally, if you can get your kid to consume 1 tablespoon of raw apple cider vinegar, do so.

The Number One Enemy of Your Child's Bowel Movements is Sugar

Children who consume too much sugar may also have diarrhea. Some sweets cause the stomach to contract, drawing out water and electrolytes and causing bowel movements to become looser. Fascinatingly, fructose, the sugar found in fruit, is the primary kind of sugar that can do this. People [or children] who consume more than 40 to 80 grams of fructose per day will get diarrhea in 75% of cases.

However, children's diarrhea may also be caused by artificial sweeteners like sorbitol or xylitol.

Suggestion
Fruit is great and contains essential vitamins, minerals, and phytochemicals, but eating too much of it may be detrimental.

Although fructose is less dangerous than sucrose, both sugars cause issues in our bloodstream when ingested in big quantities.

Teens That Consume Sugar May Have Learning Problems

According to research, youth who consume diets rich in refined sugar and saturated fat may experience brain damage, particularly to the hippocampus region of the brain, which controls memory and learning. Poor cognitive performance may result from damage to these and other brain regions caused by refined sugar and junk diet.

Suggestion

Teenagers often listen to their friends rather than their parents. If you get started as soon as possible and establish a solid rapport with them, you can alter that. When they are teenagers, if you have developed a relationship with them, they WILL listen to you. Inform children about the risks associated with consuming sugary drinks, candies, and other treats. Above all, make sure they comprehend how sugar will impact their capacity to study.

Chapter Three

Strategies for Reducing Sugar Intake in Kids

You may have seen some unwelcome withdrawal symptoms, including moodiness and tantrums if you're attempting to cut your child's sugar consumption. Children may suffer anxiety, cravings, cognitive fog, weariness, migraines, and changes in sleep habits, much like adults.

As you ingest more sugar, your body develops accustomed to its effects and needs more to produce the same high in your kid. This indicates that the cravings people feel while trying to reduce their intake of sugar might be rather strong.

Set Up A Plan

Eliminating refined sugar from your child's diet is the greatest method to help them kick their sugar habit. There are two methods to achieve this, so choose the one that works best for you and develop a strategy. Options include:

Eliminate all sugars naturally and refined for three to five days, including with fruit, starchy vegetables, and natural sweeteners like honey. After that, reintroduce fruit gradually, beginning with low-sugar alternatives like berries and starchy vegetables in moderation. Natural sweeteners should only be consumed on rare occasions. This will assist in fast ending the addiction.

Reduce your child's daily sugar intake gradually; doing so will lessen the intensity of their withdrawal symptoms, but it will take longer for them to kick the habit. With sweetened drinks, you may start lowering your sugar consumption right away. You might just dilute their drinks before switching to sugar-free options like water, depending on how severe their sugar withdrawals are. Before examining your child's natural sugar consumption, concentrate on minimizing any refined sugar-containing items they are ingesting.

Make Your Environment Cleaner

Stop purchasing items that contain refined sugar; if you keep it high up or hidden in a cabinet, it is still in their surroundings. These goods will gradually begin to make their way into your child's diet before you realize it.

Encounter Water

Encourage your kids to consume water whenever they feel hungry. We often confuse thirst with hunger, so sipping some water and waiting 10 to 15 minutes may show you are just thirsty if the hunger is under control. If switching to water is difficult, try naturally sweetening it with slices of fresh fruit like oranges or a variety of berries.

Include Healthful Fats

Avocados, nuts, seeds, and olive oil are all good sources of healthy fats that can help your child's blood sugar stay in check and keep them feeling fuller for longer. To help with satiety, a modest serving with each meal or snack will be sufficient.

Eat Normalistic Sweet vegetables

Especially when roasted, vegetables like carrots, sweet potatoes, and pumpkin have a naturally sweet flavor. This might support your kid when they experience withdrawal symptoms by satisfying their taste receptors.

Improve the Protein Quality

Quality protein will aid with satiety and blood sugar regulation, much as healthy fats do. High-quality sources of protein include quinoa, eggs, full-fat dairy products, lentils, and grass-fed beef.

Include New Foods

Focus on the things your kid can eat more of rather than the ones they can't. It may be a shock to the system, as with any diet change. Along with a change in mindset, it also calls for a change in routines and behaviors. When you are dependent on the foods that are harming you the most, this might be difficult to do.

Focusing on introducing new foods is a far more long-lasting strategy to implement change and will assist with your child's long-term sugar withdrawal symptoms. Increase your intake of protein, healthy fats, and water.

Have Your Child Activate

One of the greatest strategies to control sugar cravings is to maintain an active lifestyle. Keep in mind that exercise raises your endorphin levels, which will naturally improve your child's happiness. Walking for even 15 minutes has been shown to lessen cravings.

Encourage your kid to engage in some of their favorite activities, such as playing tag, riding a bike, or kicking a soccer ball. As a social activity, doing it with others will increase the advantages and divert attention from the sugar.

Don't Eat Any More Sugar

You should cut down on your child's sugar intake just as they are! Keep in mind that you are your child's best role model. Start becoming a good person by eating a balanced diet of whole foods.

Chapter Four

Detox for Specific Kids' Ages

Kids 1-4

Kids of this age are developing quickly, including their palates. Parents have the power to influence what their children put in their mouths, regardless of whether they are enthusiastic food explorers or picky eaters (or both on the same day). Children often prefer to have all of their meals on separate plates or in the same color scheme. Try your best to accommodate these developmental stages and encourage children to try new meals without putting any pressure on them.

For this age/stage, all detox foods are good, but you should give them extra fruit and starchy vegetables. A serving size for a kid this age should be kept in mind to be between one-third and one-half the size of an adult dish. However, children do have growth spurts during which they seem to consume indefinitely (followed by intervals during which they seem to eat very little). Provide your children with a range of sugar-free meals and let them choose how much to consume. Protein, a good fat, a starchy vegetable, and a non-starchy vegetable or fruit should all be included in every meal.

You may need to speak with the administrators if your kid attends daycare or preschool to make arrangements to bring other food for the length of the detox (or permanently). As detox programs and diets are not advised for youngsters, it is not suggested to refer to your "new" food choices as such. Furthermore, you are just giving your kid a different, sugar-free diet to help with digestion, behavior, and nutrition rather than "detoxing" them. Inform interested persons that you are going "sugar-free" if you are unsure of what else to say.

Kids 5-12

Kids in this age range go to school, dine with friends, and spend some of the day outside of their control. While it may be difficult to keep an eye on everything they eat, you may provide detox-friendly breakfasts and dinners at home and pack detox-friendly lunches and snacks for them to eat while they are out. To assist older kids comprehend how food impacts their bodies' capacity to develop normally, their minds' capacity to operate clearly, and their behavior and emotions, you may explain why you are modifying some of the things they may be consuming.

Children at this age require more carbs than adults do since they are developing, particularly as they approach puberty, much as younger children do. Build meals with the same components as your adult meals (protein, healthy fat, and vegetables) while taking into account your children's taste preferences and including starchy veggies in most of your meals. You could also wish to permit a wider range of/more portions of fruit.

Teenagers

Teenagers are nearly adults, and many of them think that they have already reached maturity, but since they are still developing, they need to eat a diet high in nutrients. However, kids may spend a lot of time away from home and may desire greater control over their food choices. If you want your adolescents to take part in the sugar detox, you should know that forcing them to do so won't be as effective as letting them choose to. If they are reluctant, you may surely remove ALL foods from the home, serve breakfasts and dinners that are suitable for a detox, and talk about how the detox is affecting your mood, ability to sleep, etc. They are becoming more independent and need to learn to make their own decisions, including those involving food, so be flexible and don't push. You are still the parent and still decide what to eat at home. Keeping the lines of communication open can help them realize that you are trying to support them in being healthy and successful in all aspects of their life. You may also need to embrace the possibility that they may overindulge in sugary foods when at school or friends' homes.

At this time, I would still provide starchy carbs to teenagers at least once a day, preferably more, if they are particularly active or between the ages of 13 and 16 (about). As they go through development spurts, infants may even consume larger meals than adults. But as they age, their development will ultimately halt, and they won't need as much fruit or starchy food to keep their energy levels up and their capacity to expand. Watch them carefully, however, and if you see significant changes in their sleep, behavior, or energy levels, give them additional rich carbohydrates. Even studying demands a significant amount of energy!

Chapter Five

Sugar Detox Meal Plan for Kids

Day 1

Breakfast

Fried eggs with avocado and spinach

Snacks

Apple slices with almond butter

Lunch

Lettuce wraps with turkey and cheese and

cherry tomatoes

Snack

Hummus and carrot sticks

Dinner

Roasted broccoli, sweet potato wedges, and

baked chicken

Day 2

Breakfast

Greek yogurt and berries on top of oatmeal

Snack

Cream cheese-topped celery sticks

Lunch

Grilled chicken Caesar salad

Snack

Hard-boiled egg

Dinner

Baked salmon with quinoa and asparagus

Day 3

Breakfast

Chia seed pudding with banana and cinnamon

Snack

Cucumber slices with tzatziki sauce

Lunch

Veggie-packed turkey chili

Snack

Munchies Homemade popcorn

Dinner

Zucchini noodles with marinara and turkey meatballs

Day 4

Breakfast

Banana slices with almond butter on whole-grain bread

Snack

Guacamole with bell pepper slices

Lunch

Skewers of grilled chicken and vegetables

Snack

Cheese stick with grapes

Dinner

Filled baked sweet potato with meat and vegetables

Day 5

Breakfast

Greek yogurt with mixed berries and honey

Snack

Hard-boiled egg

Lunch

Salad with tomatoes, cheese, and balsamic vinaigrette

Snack

Raw almonds

Dinner

Brown rice with grilled shrimp with roasted Brussels sprouts

Day 6

Breakfast

Black beans, salsa, and tortilla with scrambled

eggs

Snack

Smoothie with banana and almond butter.

Lunch

Brown rice, green beans, and roasted turkey

breast

Snack

Cherry tomatoes with mozzarella cheese

Dinner

Stir-fried beef with bell peppers, broccoli, and

brown rice

Day 7

Breakfast

Greek yogurt with granola and fresh fruit

Sugar Detox Diet Recipes for Kids

Snack

Raw vegetables with ranch dressing

Lunch

Cucumber slices and tuna salad in lettuce cups

Snack

Fresh berries with whipped cream

Dinner

Roasted sweet potatoes, roasted green beans,

and baked chicken

View the recipes' preparation method here:

Scrambled Eggs with Avocado and Spinach

Ingredients:

2 eggs

Fresh spinach, half a cup

Sliced avocado, half

Olive oil, 1 tbsp

Pepper and salt as desired

Prep Time: 10 minutes

Method

- Over medium heat, warm the olive oil.

- For 1-2 minutes, add the spinach and cook until wilted.

- When the eggs are fully cooked, scramble them in the pan.

- Add the cubed avocado and taste-test your seasoning with salt and pepper.

- Enjoy a hot serving.

Slices of Apple with Almond Butter

Ingredients:

2 tablespoons of almond butter

1 medium-sized apple, sliced

Prep time: 5 minutes

Method

- Cut the apple into paper-thin slices.

- Each slice should have almond butter applied to it.
- Enjoy after serving.

Lettuce Wraps with Cherry Tomatoes and Turkey and Cheese

Ingredients:

4 big leaves of lettuce

4 turkey breast slices

4 cheese slices

Halved 8 cherry tomatoes

Prep time: 10 minutes

Method

- Set the lettuce leaves out.
- Each lettuce leaf should include a piece of cheese and a slice of turkey.
- Cherry tomatoes may be added on top.
- Serve the lettuce leaves rolled up.

Hummus with Carrot Sticks

Ingredients:

Cut two big carrots into sticks.

¼ cup of hummus

Prep time: 5 minutes

Method

- Sticks of carrots should be cut.
- Serve as a dip with hummus.

Sweet Potato Wedges, Roasted Broccoli, and Baked Chicken

Ingredients:

2 breasts of chicken

2 cups of florets from broccoli

Wedges sliced from 2 medium-sized sweet potatoes

Olive oil, 2 tablespoons

Pepper and salt as desired

Prep time:30 minutes

Method

- Set the oven's temperature to 400°F (200°C).
- Chicken breasts should be salted and peppered.
- On a baking sheet, put the chicken breasts and bake them for 20 to 25 minutes, or until done.
- Olive oil, salt, and pepper should be tossed with the slices of broccoli and sweet potato.
- On a separate baking sheet, arrange the broccoli and sweet potato wedges, and roast for 20 to 25 minutes, or until soft.
- Enjoy a hot serving.

Oatmeal with Berries and a Dollop of Greek Yogurt

Ingredients:

Rollin oats in a cup, half

1 cup of milk or water

Strawberries, blueberries, and raspberries make up half a cup of mixed berries.

1/4 cup of Greek yogurt

Prep time: 10 minutes

Method

- Bring the oats, water, and milk to a boil in a saucepan.
- Stirring periodically, lower the heat, and simmer for 5-7 minutes.
- Place the oats in a bowl and top with a dollop of Greek yogurt and the mixed berries.
- Enjoy a hot serving.

Cream Cheese with Celery Sticks

Ingredients:

4 sticks of celery

Cream cheese, two teaspoons

Prep time: 5 minutes

Method

- Make 4-inch-long chunks out of the celery sticks.
- Cream cheese is stuffed within the celery.
- Enjoy after serving.

Salad with Grilled Chicken Caesar

Ingredients:

2 skinless, boneless breasts of chicken

4 cups of chopped Romaine lettuce

Caesar dressing, 1/4 cup

Grated Parmesan cheese, 1/4 cup

Prep time: 30 minutes

Method

- Set the grill's temperature to medium-high.
- Chicken breasts should be salted and peppered.

- The chicken breasts should be cooked through, about 6 to 8 minutes each side.
- Let the chicken breasts cool off before slicing..
- The chopped Romaine lettuce, Caesar dressing, and Parmesan cheese should all be combined in a big dish.
- Place the chicken slices on top.
- Serve after tossing the salad.

Quinoa, Asparagus, and Baked Salmon

Ingredients:

2 filets of salmon

1 kilogram of asparagus

One cup quinoa

Olive oil, 2 tablespoons

Pepper and salt as desired

Prep time: 40 minutes

Method

- Set the oven's temperature to 400°F (200°C).
- To prepare the quinoa, follow the directions on the box.
- Brush some olive oil on a baking pan and add the salmon filets.
- Add salt and pepper to taste.
- On a different baking sheet, arrange the asparagus and sprinkle it with olive oil.
- Add salt and pepper to taste.
- For 15 to 20 minutes, roast the salmon and asparagus in the oven, or until they are soft.
- Along with the cooked quinoa, serve the salmon and asparagus.

Chia Seed Pudding with Banana and Cinnamon

Ingredients:

1 mashed ripe banana

1 cup of almond milk without sugar

Chia seeds, 1/4 cup

1 teaspoon of cinnamon

Honey or maple syrup for sweetness (optional)

Prep time: 5 minutes plus one night of cooling

Method

- Banana puree, almond milk, chia seeds, and cinnamon should all be combined in a mixing dish.

- Stir everything together well. If you'd like, taste and add more honey or maple syrup.

- Keep overnight in the refrigerator, and cover the bowl.

- Stir the ingredients and portion them into serving dishes or jars in the morning.

- If preferred, garnish with chopped nuts, sliced bananas, or fresh berries.

Cucumber Slices with Tzatziki Sauce

Ingredients:

Sliced big cucumber, 1

Greek yogurt, plain, in 1/2 cup

Fresh dill, cut into 1/4 cup

1 minced clove of garlic,

1 tablespoon lemon juice

To taste, add salt and black pepper.

Process time: 10 minutes

Method

- Combine Greek yogurt, dill, garlic, and lemon juice in a small mixing basin.
- Add salt and black pepper after thoroughly combining.
- Sliced cucumber should be served with tzatziki sauce on the side.

Turkey Chili with Vegetables

Ingredients:

1 pound of turkey meat

1 chopped onion

2 minced garlic cloves

1 diced bell pepper

1 diced zucchini

1 can (15 oz) of kidney beans

1 can (15 oz) shredded tomatoes

1.5 tbsp cumin powder

1 teaspoon cumin

To taste, add salt and black pepper.

Optional garnishes: diced avocado, shredded cheese, and chopped cilantro

Prep time: 15 minutes

Method

- A little drizzle of olive oil should be heated over medium-high heat in a big saucepan or Dutch oven.

- When browned, add the ground turkey and cook it while breaking it up with a spoon.

- Add zucchini, bell pepper, onion, and garlic to the saucepan. Cook until they are tender.

- To the saucepan, add kidney beans, chopped tomatoes, cumin, chili powder, salt, and black pepper. To blend, thoroughly stir.
- The mixture should simmer for 20 to 25 minutes while being intermittently stirred.
- Serve hot with any preferred garnishes.

Homemade Popcorn

Ingredients:

1/4 cup kernels of popcorn

2 tbsp. of olive oil

To taste, sea salt

Prep time: 5 minutes

Method

- Olive oil should be heated over medium-high heat in a big saucepan with a cover.

- Popcorn kernels should be added to the pot before the lid is on.
- Occasionally shake the pot to avoid scorching the kernels.
- Remove the saucepan from the heat when the popping calms down.
- Add sea salt to taste and place the popcorn in a big bowl.

Marinara Sauce over Zucchini Noodles with Turkey Meatballs

Ingredients:

1 pound of turkey meat

A half-cup of almond flour

1 egg

2 minced garlic cloves

1 tbsp. freshly chopped parsley

To taste, add salt and black pepper.

Two substantial zucchini, spiralized

1 cup of sauce for pasta

Optional garnishes: parmesan cheese, grated

Prep time: 20 minutes

Method

- Ground turkey, almond flour, egg, garlic, parsley, salt, and black pepper should all be combined in a mixing bowl.
- Mix well and shape into little meatballs using your hands.
- In a big skillet, warm up some olive oil over medium-high heat.
- The meatballs should be added to the pan and cooked for 8 to 10 minutes, turning them over halfway through, until browned and well done.
- Put the meatballs aside, when it is done
- In the same pan, add the spiralized zucchini and cook for 2 to 3 minutes, or until tender.
- Stir the zucchini noodles and marinara sauce together in a pan.

- Reintroduce the meatballs to the pan and boil the mixture for an additional five minutes.
- Serve hot with any preferred garnishes.

Sliced Banana and Whole-grain Toast with Almond Butter

Ingredients:

A pair of whole-grain bread slices

2/butter almonds

Sliced banana, one

Prep time: 5 minutes

Method

- In a toaster, toast the whole-grain bread.
- Each piece of bread should have 1 tablespoon of almond butter on it.
- A sliced banana is placed on top of each slice.

Bell Pepper Slices with Guacamole

Ingredients:

1 sliced bell pepper

1 mature avocado

Tomato dice, 1/4 cup

Onion, diced, 1/4 cup

10 ml of lime juice

To taste, add salt and black pepper.

Prep time: 10 minutes

Method

- Slice the bell pepper and put it aside.

- Use a fork to mash the avocado in a small mixing basin.

- To the bowl, add the chopped tomatoes, onion, lime juice, salt, and black pepper. Mix thoroughly.

Guacamole should be served with bell pepper slices.

Grilled Chicken and Vegetable Skewers

Ingredients :

1 pound of cubed, skinless, boneless chicken breast

1 Sliced zucchini

Cut one red onion into wedges.

A single red bell pepper, diced

One yellow bell pepper, diced

2 tbsp. of olive oil

Dry thyme, 1 teaspoon

To taste, add salt and black pepper.

Prep time: 20 minutes

Method

- Grill at a medium-high temperature.
- Skewers are topped with chicken, zucchini, red onion, red bell pepper, and yellow bell pepper.
- Combine the olive oil, salt, black pepper, and dried thyme in a small mixing bowl.

- Apply the olive oil mixture on the skewers.
- The skewers should be cooked through and slightly browned after 8 to 10 minutes of grilling, rotating them once or twice.
- Serve warm.

Cheese Sticks and Grapes

Ingredients:

One cheese stick

A few grapes

Prep time: 2 minutes

Method

- Cheese sticks should be cut into pieces.
- Grapes on the side should be served with the cheese slices.

Ground Beef and Vegetables Stuffed in a Baked Sweet Potato

Ingredients:

Two large sweet potatoes

1/2 pound of ground beef

1/2 cup chopped bell pepper

1/2 cup diced onion

chopped zucchini, half a cup

Dried oregano, 1 teaspoon

To taste, add salt and black pepper.

Prep time: 15 minutes

Method

- Set the oven to 400°F.
- The sweet potatoes should be washed and punched many times with a fork.
- Bake the sweet potatoes for 40–45 minutes, or until they are soft, on a baking sheet.
- Warm up a generous amount of olive oil in a big pan over medium-high heat while the sweet potatoes are roasting.

- Add salt, black pepper, dried oregano, onion, bell pepper, zucchini, and ground beef to the skillet. Cook the veggies and meat until they are tender.

- Allow the sweet potatoes to cool when they are finished cooking.

- Cut them in half lengthwise, then hollow out a portion of the meat.

- The ground beef and vegetable combination should be placed into each sweet potato half.

- Bake the filled sweet potatoes once more in the oven.

Greek Yogurt with a Variety of Berries and Honey Drizzle

Ingredients:

1 cup of Greek yogurt, plain

Strawberries, blueberries, and raspberries totaling 1/2 cup

1 teaspoon of honey

Prep time: 5 minutes

Method

- Greek yogurt should be poured into a bowl.
- Add a mixture of berries to the yogurt.
- Honey should be drizzled on top.
- Offer chilled.

Salad with Tomatoes and Mozzarella with Balsamic Vinaigrette

Ingredients:

4 ounces of fresh mozzarella cheese

Cut into two, medium-sized tomatoes

Balsamic vinegar, 1 tablespoon

1 tablespoon of olive oil

Dijon mustard, 1 teaspoon

To taste, add salt and black pepper.

Prep time: 10 minutes

Method

- Place the mozzarella cheese and tomato slices on a platter.
- Balsamic vinegar, olive oil, Dijon mustard, salt, and black pepper should be combined in a small mixing dish.
- Over the salad, drizzle the balsamic vinaigrette.
- Offer chilled.

Brown Rice with Grilled Shrimp with Roasted Brussels Sprouts

Ingredients:

Peeled, and deveined shrimp, 1 pound

Trimmed and halved Brussels sprouts, one pound

2 tbsp. of olive oil

Garlic powder, 1 teaspoon

To taste, add salt and black pepper.

2 cups of brown rice, cooked

Prep time: 20 minutes

Method

- Grill at a medium-high temperature.

- Toss the shrimp with 1 tablespoon of olive oil and garlic powder in a mixing bowl. Place aside.

- Toss the Brussels sprouts with 1 tablespoon of olive oil, salt, and black pepper on a baking sheet.

- For 15 to 20 minutes, roast the Brussels sprouts at 400°F in the oven, or until they are soft and gently browned.

- Grill the shrimp for 2 to 3 minutes on each side, or until pink and just starting to brown.

- Over a bed of cooked brown rice, plate the roasted Brussels sprouts and grilled shrimp.

Scrambled Eggs, Black beans, and Salsa in a Burrito

Ingredients:

Two huge eggs

1/4 cup washed and drained black beans

Salsa, two tablespoons

1 tortilla whole-wheat

Prep time: 10 minutes

Method

- In a small dish, crack the eggs and mix them.
- The eggs are added to a non-stick skillet that is already hot. Cook the scramble thoroughly.
- Either in the microwave or on the stove, reheat the black beans.
- The tortilla should be warmed all the way through in the microwave or on the stove.

- Place the black beans and scrambled eggs in the tortilla's middle.
- Place Salsa on top, wrap the tortilla, and eat!

Smoothie with Almond Butter and Bananas

Ingredients:

One ripe banana

1/4 cup almond butter

1 cup of almond milk without sugar

1/8 teaspoon of cinnamon powder

A smidge of vanilla extract

Prep time: 5 minutes

Method

- Put all ingredients in a blender, then blend until they are smooth.
- Serve right away and enjoy!

Brown Rice, Green Beans, and Roasted Turkey Breast

Ingredients:

Roasted turkey breast, 4 oz.

1 cup trimmed green beans

boiled according to package instructions

Half a cup of brown rice

Olive oil, 1 tbsp

Pepper and salt as desired

Prep time: 20 minutes

Method

- Set the oven's temperature to 400°F (200°C).
- Bake the turkey breast for 15 to 20 minutes, or until it is well done.
- In another dish, toss the green beans with the olive oil, salt, and pepper.
- Put the brown rice and green beans on a platter.

- Rice and green beans are served with sliced turkey breast on top.

Cherry Tomatoes and Mozzarella Cheese

Ingredients:

Cherry tomatoes, 1 cup

2 ounces of sliced fresh mozzarella cheese

¼ cup balsamic vinegar

Olive oil, 1 tbsp

Pepper and salt as desired

5 minutes to prepare

Method

- Cherry tomatoes should be washed and cut in half.
- On a platter, arrange the mozzarella cheese and tomatoes.
- Olive oil and balsamic vinegar should be drizzled on.
- To taste, add salt and pepper.

Brown Rice, Broccoli, and Beef Stir-fried

Ingredients:

4 ounces of thinly sliced lean beef

broccoli florets in a cup

Sliced bell peppers in a cup

boiled according to package instructions

Half a cup of brown rice

Olive oil, 1 tbsp

Low-sodium soy sauce, 1 tbsp

1 teaspoon of powdered garlic

Prep time: 20 minutes

Method

- In a big skillet or wok, heat the olive oil over high heat.
- Stir-fry the beef for two to three minutes, or until it is browned on both sides.
- When the veggies are tender-crisp, add the broccoli and bell peppers to the pan and stir-fry for an additional two to three minutes.

- Stir the soy sauce and garlic powder together in the skillet.
- Serve brown rice with the meat stir-fry.

Granola and Fresh Fruit with Greek Yogurt

Ingredients:

Greek yogurt, one cup

1/4 cup of cereal

1/2 cup of assorted fresh fruit, such as berries, banana slices, or apple chunks

Prep time: 5 minutes

Method

- Combine the Greek yogurt and granola in a small bowl.
- Enjoy! Add some fresh fruit on top.

Raw Vegetables with Ranch Dressing

Ingredients:

1 cup of raw vegetables, such as cherry tomatoes, cucumber slices, carrot sticks, and bell pepper strips

1/4 cup of unsweetened Greek yogurt

1/9 cup dried parsley

One tablespoon of dried dill

1 teaspoon of powdered garlic

One-half teaspoon of onion powder

Pepper and salt as desired

Prep time: 10 minutes

Method

- Your vegetables should be washed, cut into bite-sized pieces, and placed on a platter.

- Greek yogurt, dried herbs, garlic powder, onion powder, salt, and pepper should all be well blended in a small dish with Greek yogurt.

- Ranch dip should be served with the vegetables for dipping.

Tuna Salad with Cucumber Slices and Lettuce

Ingredients:

1 can of drained tuna

Greek yogurt, plain, two teaspoons

1/9 cup Dijon mustard

One teaspoon of lemon juice

Pepper and salt as desired

Lettuce leaves (such as romaine or butter lettuce)

Cucumber slices for serving

Prep time: 10 minutes

Method

- Tuna, Greek yogurt, Dijon mustard, lemon juice, salt, and pepper should all be well mixed in a medium bowl.
- Fill the lettuce cups with the tuna salad.

- Cucumber slices should be served on the side.

Whipped Cream with Fresh Berries

Ingredients:

1 cup of fresh berries, using a mixture of strawberries, blueberries, and raspberries

50 ml of thick cream

1 tablespoon of sugar, powder

One-half teaspoon of vanilla extract

Prep time: 10 minutes

Method

- The berries should be washed, chopped, and put on a platter.
- Use an electric mixer to whisk the heavy cream in a medium bowl until firm peaks form.
- Until well blended, fold in the powdered sugar and vanilla essence.

- Berries should be placed on the side with the whipped cream.

Roasted Sweet Potatoes, Green Beans, and Baked Chicken

Ingredients:

2 skinless, boneless breasts of chicken

2 chopped and peeled sweet potatoes

1 pound of trimmed green beans

Olive oil, two teaspoons

pepper and salt as desired

Prep time: 15 minutes

Method

- Set the oven's temperature to 400°F (200°C).

- Add salt and pepper to the chicken breasts before placing them in a baking tray.

- In another dish, toss the green beans and sweet potatoes with the olive oil, salt, and pepper.
- Place the chicken in the baking dish and surround it with the sweet potatoes and green beans.
- Bake for 30 minutes, or until the chicken is cooked enough, and the veggies are soft.

Even with meals that look healthy, such as yogurt and granola bars, pay attention to product labels and minimize added sugars.

Chapter Six

Kids Recipes for a Sugar Detox

Children's Menu Options

Rethinking your food choices while beginning a sugar detox may be extremely difficult, particularly if you are accustomed to consuming a lot of refined grain goods or sweet desserts. Finding kid-friendly foods for sugar detox might be even harder. You may discover some kid-friendly solutions below.

Beverages suitable for kids

- Coconut Juice
- If your kids eat dairy products and have access to raw cow's milk
- Sparkling water

- Herbal tea (often served chilled; favorites include peppermint and unsweetened fruity varieties)
- Light coconut milk is more appetizing as a beverage.
- Kombucha (try Diane's recipe for homemade Kombucha)
- Smoothies

Child-friendly snacks

- Raw veggies with guacamole, classic hummus, or cauliflower.
- Celery or a green apple with nut butter
- Coconut-flour biscuits or muffins
- Smoothies—try one like this: organic plain full-fat yogurt with cinnamon, apple, or banana
- Sugar-free jerky beef
- Whole seeds and nuts
- Nut mix or granola without grains

- Sandwich meat rolls

- Olives

- Sweet potatoes steamed

- Fried sweet potatoes

- (Coconut oil-fried) plantain chips,

(If they tolerate dairy products well)

- Truffles with coconut butter or lemon vanilla meltaways

- Pumpkin, almond, or coconut flour pancakes

- Flakes of toasted coconut

- Burnt seaweed

Regardless of what you consume! When necessary, modify preparation and portion sizes.

Breakfast Ideas

Banana-Oatmeal Pancakes

Ingredients:

One ripe banana

Oats, rolled, in a cup

half a teaspoon of cinnamon

A half-teaspoon of baking powder

1/4 teaspoon salt

1/4 cup unsweetened milk

1 egg

Prep time: 10 minutes

Method

- Bananas are prepared by being mashed in a bowl.
- Add the milk, egg, baking powder, salt, oats, and cinnamon. Stir everything together.
- On a medium heat, place the nonstick skillet.

- Pour a quarter cup of the batter into the skillet, for each pancake.
- Leave until it is brown, 2 to 3 minutes on each side.
- Include fruit while serving.

Avocado Toast

Ingredients:

1 slice whole grain bread

1/2 ripe avocado.

Pepper and salt

Fresh lemon juice squeezed

Prep time: 5 minutes

Method

- Toast the bread as a preparation technique.
- Mash the avocado in a small bowl.
- Toast is covered with mashed avocado.
- Add salt and pepper to taste.
- Add some freshly squeezed lemon juice.

- Serve with fresh fruit or a hard-boiled egg.

Sweet Potato Hash

Ingredients:

1 sweet potato, diced after peeling

1/2 onion

1 red bell pepper, diced after peeling

2 cloves minced

2 tablespoons of olive oil.

Pepper and salt as desired

Prep time: 15 minutes

Method

- Over medium heat, warm the olive oil in a pan
- Add the red bell pepper, onion, and sweet potato. The sweet potato should be cooked for 10 to 12 minutes, stirring periodically, until it is soft.

- For a further one to two minutes, add the garlic.
- Add salt and pepper to the food.
- Serve with turkey sausage or scrambled eggs.

Parfait of Greek yogurt

Ingredients:

1 cup of Greek yogurt, plain

A half-cup of fresh berries

1/4 cup of cereal

1 tablespoon of optional honey

Prep time: 5 minutes

Method

- In a dish or container, arrange the yogurt, berries, and granola in layers.
- If desired, drizzle with honey.
- Offer chilled.

Veggie Egg Scramble

Ingredients:

Two eggs

1/4 cup of bell peppers, diced

chopped zucchini

1/4 cup sliced onion

Pepper and salt as desired

Olive oil, 1 tbsp

Prep time: 10 minutes

Method

- Olive oil is heated in a pan over medium heat during preparation.
- Add the onion, zucchini, and bell peppers. Cook until tender for 5-7 minutes.
- Whisk eggs in a bowl, before being added to the skillet.
- When the eggs are set, cook for another 2-3 minutes, stirring periodically.
- Add salt and pepper to the food.

- With whole grain toast, serve.

Made-at-Home Granola Bars

Ingredients:

1/4 cup chopped nuts (almonds, pecans, etc.)

1/2 cup rolled oats.

1/4 cup coconut shreds without sugar

1/4 cup of raisins and cranberries, dried fruit

1/4 cup natural almond or peanut butter

1/4 cup honey and 1/fourth teaspoon vanilla essence

A dash of salt

Prep time: 20 minutes

Method

- The oven should be preheated at 350°F (175°C).
- Line a baking sheet with a parchment paper.

- The dried fruit, nuts, shredded coconut, and oats should all be combined in a large mixing dish.
- The peanut or almond butter, honey, vanilla extract, and salt should all be combined until smooth in a different mixing dish.
- Mix the dry ingredients first, then add the peanut or almond butter combination.
- Spread out evenly after transferring the mixture to the prepared baking dish.
- Bake for 25 minutes, or until golden.
- Before cutting into bars, let stand for 10 to 15 minutes to cool.
- Serve with yogurt or fresh fruit.

Smoothie Verde

Ingredients:

1 cup of kale or spinach

One ripe banana

A half-cup of frozen berries

1/2 cup almond milk without sugar

1/4 cup of unsweetened Greek yogurt

Chia seeds, one tablespoon

Prep time: 5 minutes

Method

- All components should be combined in a blender and blended until smooth.
- If necessary, add additional almond milk to get the required consistency.
- Offer chilled.

Apple Cinnamon Quinoa Bowl

Ingredients:

1 cup cooked quinoa

1/2 cup unsweetened applesauce

Chopped walnuts, 1/4 cup

Half a teaspoon of cinnamon

1 tablespoon of optional honey

Prep time: 10 minutes

Method

- In a bowl, mix the quinoa, applesauce, walnuts, and cinnamon.
- If desired, drizzle with honey.
- Serve hot.

Egg and Veggie Muffins

Ingredients:

6 eggs

Vegetables, such as spinach, bell peppers, mushrooms, etc., totaling 1/2 cup

Pepper and salt as desired

Prep time: 20 minutes

Method

- Set the oven's temperature to 350°F (175°C).
- Use nonstick spray to grease a muffin pan.
- Whisk the eggs in a bowl

- Add the chopped vegetables and salt & pepper to taste.
- Fill each muffin cup to the top equally with the egg mixture.
- Bake the eggs for 15 to 20 minutes, or until they are set.
- Before removing them from the muffin tray, let them cool for a few minutes.
- Serve with fresh fruit or whole-grain bread.

Chia Seed Dessert

Ingredients:

¼ cup of Chia seeds

1 cup of almond milk without sugar

1 teaspoon of honey

One-half teaspoon of vanilla extract

Prep time: 5 minutes

Method

- In a bowl, combine all the ingredients and whisk thoroughly.

- Allowing the mixture to thicken will take 10 to 15 minutes.

- Serve chilled with sliced bananas or fresh berries.

Lunch and Dinner Recipes

Skewers of Grilled Chicken and Vegetables

Ingredients:

1 pound of cubed, skinless, boneless chicken breasts

Two bell peppers, chopped

One red onion, chopped

A single zucchini, chopped

1 tablespoon of olive oil

To taste salt and pepper

Prep time: 20 minutes

Method

- Prepare by heating the grill to a medium-high temperature.
- Skewers with veggies and chicken should be used.
- Olive oil should be used, then salt and pepper should be added.
- Until the chicken is well cooked and the veggies are soft, grill the skewers for 10 to 15 minutes, rotating them once.
- Serve with quinoa or full-grain rice.

Soup with Lentils and Veggies

Ingredients:

Olive oil, one tablespoon

1 onion, minced

2 garlic cloves

2 carrots

2 celery stalks

1 red bell pepper

1 can of diced tomatoes

1 cup washed red lentils

1 teaspoon cumin to 4 cups of vegetable broth

Smoked paprika, 1/2 teaspoon

Pepper and salt as desired

Prep time: 10 minutes

Method

- Olive oil is heated in a big saucepan over medium heat during preparation.

- Sauté the garlic and omion until tender.

- Cook the carrots, celery, and bell pepper for a further five minutes.

- Cumin, smoked paprika, salt, pepper, lentils, chopped tomatoes, and vegetable broth should all be stirred in.

- When the lentils are ready, bring to a boil, then lower the heat and simmer for 20 to 25 minutes.

- Serve hot with whole-grain bread on the side.

Bowl of Black Beans and Quinoa

Ingredients:

One cup of cooked quinoa is included.

A can of Black beans rinsed and drained black beans

1 chopped red bell pepper

1 diced avocado

1/4 cup finely minced fresh cilantro

1 juiced lime

Pepper and salt as desired

Prep time: 10 minutes

Method

- Quinoa, black beans, red bell pepper, avocado, cilantro, lime juice, salt, and pepper are combined in a mixing bowl as the preparation method.

- Mix well by tossing, at room temperature or chilly.

Baked Sweet Potato Fries

Ingredients:

Peel and cut into fries, two sweet potatoes

1 tablespoon of olive oil

1 teaspoon paprika

1/2 teaspoon of garlic powder

Pepper and salt as desired

Prep time: 10 minutes

Method

- The oven should be preheated to 425°F (220°C).

- Cover the baking sheet with parchment paper.

- Fries made from sweet potatoes should be mixed with olive oil, salt, pepper, paprika, and garlic powder.

- Fries should be arranged on the baking pan in one layer.

- Bake fries until crispy and golden brown for 20 to 25 minutes, turning halfway through.
- Serve hot with a Greek yogurt dip on the side.

Veggie and Bean Burrito Bowl

Ingredients:

1 cup of brown rice, cooked

Rinsed and drained can of Black beans

1 chopped red bell pepper

1 diced avocado

1/4 cup finely minced fresh cilantro

1 juiced lime

Pepper and salt as desired

Prep time: 10 minutes

Method

- Brown rice, black beans, red bell pepper, avocado, cilantro, lime juice, salt, and pepper should all be combined in a mixing dish.

- Mix well by tossing, at room temperature or chilly.

Stir-fried Vegetables and Chicken

Ingredients:

Skinless and boneless chicken breasts, sliced into strips, a pound

Two cups of mixed veggies, such as broccoli, carrots, and snap peas

2 minced garlic cloves

1 teaspoon ginger

1 tablespoon of olive oil

1/9 cup soy sauce

Pepper and salt as desired

Prep time: 15 minutes

Method

- Olive oil is heated in a large pan or wok over medium-high heat during preparation.
- Add the chicken and stir-fry for 5 to 7 minutes, or until cooked through.
- Stir-fry for an additional 5-7 minutes, or until the veggies are soft, after which you add the mixed vegetables, garlic, ginger, soy sauce, salt, and pepper.
- Serve hot with a serving of quinoa or brown rice.

Vegetable and Tuna Salad

Ingredients

2 cans of drained tuna in water

2 cups greens for a mixed salad

Sliced cucumber, bell pepper, avocado, 1 tablespoon of olive oil

1-tablespoon lemon juice

Pepper and salt as desired

Prep time: p10 minutes

Method

- Tuna, salad greens, cucumber, bell pepper, avocado, olive oil, lemon juice, salt, and pepper should all be combined in a mixing dish.
- Mix well by tossing.
- Offer chilled.

Noodles with Tomato Sauce and Zucchini

Ingredients:

Two substantial zucchini, spiralized

1 chopped onion

2 minced garlic cloves

1 tomato-diced can

Dried oregano, 1 teaspoon

½ teaspoon dried basil

pepper and salt as desired

Prep time: 10 minutes

Method

- Olive oil is heated in a large pan over medium heat during preparation.
- Sauté the garlic and onion until tender.
- Add salt, pepper, oregano, basil, and chopped tomatoes.
- Simmer the sauce for 10 to 15 minutes, or until it thickens.
- Zucchini noodles should be cooked for 5-7 minutes in olive oil in a separate pan.
- Tomato sauce over top and serve hot.

Chili with Sweet Potatoes and Black Beans

Ingredients:

Olive oil, one tablespoon

1 diced onion

2 minced garlic cloves

2 chopped and peeled sweet potatoes

1 can of black beans, rinsed and drained

1 tomato-diced can

1 teaspoon of chili powder in 2 cups of
vegetable broth

1/2 teaspoon cumin

Pepper and salt as desired

10 minutes for preparation

Time to cook: 25–30 minutes

Method

- In a big saucepan, warm up the olive oil over medium heat.
- Stir in the onion and garlic, cooking until tender.
- Add the vegetable broth, cumin, salt, pepper, chili powder, black beans, chopped tomatoes, and sweet potatoes.
- Bring to a boil, then lower the heat and simmer the sweet potatoes for 20 to 25 minutes, or until they are fork-tender.
- Serve hot with an avocado or dollop of plain Greek yogurt on top.

Stir-fry Vegetables with Quinoa

Ingredients:

One cup of cooked quinoa

Two cups of mixed veggies, such as broccoli, carrots, and snap peas

2 minced garlic cloves

1 teaspoon ginger

1 tablespoon of olive oil

1/9 cup soy sauce

Pepper and salt as desired

Prep time: 10 minutes

Method

- Heat the olive oil over medium-high heat.
- Stir-fry the veggies for 5-7 minutes, or until they are soft, adding the garlic, ginger, soy sauce, salt, and pepper as needed.

- Stir-fry the cooked quinoa for an additional two to three minutes, or until it is well-heated.
- Serve warm.

Foil Packets with Vegetables and Salmon

Ingredients:

2 filets of salmon

Two cups of mixed veggies, such as broccoli, carrots, and snap peas

1 sliced lemon

2 tbsp. of olive oil

Pepper and salt as desired

Prep time: 10 minutes

Method

- Preparation procedure: Heat the oven to 400°F (200°C).
- Salmon filets should be placed on a big piece of aluminum foil.

- Salmon should be surrounded by mixed veggies and lemon slices.
- Add salt and pepper to taste
- Sprinkle with olive oil.
- To make a sealed pouch, fold the foil over the salmon and veggies.
- Once the salmon is cooked through and the veggies are soft, place the package on a baking tray and bake for 15-20 minutes.
- Serve warm.

Soup with Lentils and Veggies

Ingredients:

Olive oil, one tablespoon

1 cup dry lentils, washed and drained,

1 onion, diced

2 garlic cloves, minced

2 carrots, diced

2 celery stalks, diced.

1 teaspoon dried thyme in 4 cups of vegetable broth

Pepper and salt as desired

Prep time: 10 minutes

Method

- In a big saucepan, warm up the olive oil over medium heat.
- Sauté the garlics and onion until tender.
- Cook the carrots and celery after adding them for 5-7 minutes, or until they are soft.
- Bring to a boil the lentils, vegetable broth, thyme, salt, and pepper.
- Reduce heat and simmer lentils for 25–30 minutes, or until they are cooked through.
- Serve hot with whole-grain bread on the side.

Vegetable Frittata

Ingredients:

6 eggs

½ cup of finely chopped mixed vegetables, such as spinach and bell peppers.

1/4 cup feta cheese crumbles

1 tablespoon of olive oil

Pepper and salt as desired

Prep time: 10 minutes

Method

- Set the oven's temperature to 350°F (180°C).

- Beat eggs, salt, and pepper together in a big basin.

- In a large oven-safe skillet, warm olive oil over medium heat.

- For 5-7 minutes, or until the veggies are soft, add the mixed vegetables.

- The edges should start to set after two to three minutes of cooking the egg mixture in the pan.

- Feta cheese should be added on top.

- Bake the frittata for 8 to 10 minutes, or until it is fully cooked through and golden on top, in the preheated oven.

- Serve hot or at room temperature after cutting into wedges.

Note: These recipes may be modified to suit your child's preferences and nutritional needs. Before making any big dietary changes for your kid, always speak with a healthcare professional or certified dietician.

Healthy Snacks

Sandwiches with Apple and Almond Butter

Ingredients:

Round slices of one apple

2 butter almonds

A tbsp of chia seeds

Prep time: 5 minutes

Method

- Each apple round should have almond butter applied on one side.
- One apple round should have chia seeds on top of it.
- Place the second apple round on top with the sides that contain the almond butter facing one another.
- Gently press down to create a sandwich.

Roasted Chickpeas

Ingredients:

1 can of washed and drained chickpeas.

1 teaspoon olive oil

1/2 teaspoon of garlic powder

Paprika, 1/2 tsp.

Salt as desired

Prep time: 5 minutes

Method

- Preparation procedure: Heat the oven to 400°F (200°C).

- Using a paper towel, dry the chickpeas.

- Chickpeas should be combined with salt, paprika, garlic powder, and olive oil in a bowl.

- On a baking sheet, spread the chickpeas out in a single layer.

- Roast for 20 to 25 minutes, or until crispy, in the preheated oven.

- Store in an airtight container after allowing it to cool.

Carrot and Hummus Dipper Sticks

Ingredients :

2 big carrots, peeled and sliced into sticks

2 tablespoons of hummus

Prep time: 5 minutes

Method

- Prepare by arranging carrot sticks on a platter.
- For dipping, put the hummus in a small bowl.

Yogurt Berry Parfait

Ingredients:

1 cup of Greek yogurt, plain

Strawberries, blueberries, and raspberries totaling 1/2 cup

1 tablespoon of honey

1/4 cup of cereal

Prep time: 5 minutes

Method

- In a glass or dish, layer yogurt, berries, and granola for preparation.
- On top, drizzle honey.

Cucumber and Cream Cheese Bites

Ingredients:

1 cucumber, cut into rounds.

2 batches of cream cheese

1-teaspoon dried dill

Prep time: 5 minutes

Method

- Spread cream cheese on one side of each cucumber round during preparation.
- On top of the cream cheese, scatter some dill.
- Offer chilled.

Chocolate Avocado Pudding

Ingredients:

1 ripe avocado

cocoa powder, 1/4 cup

½ batch of maple syrup

¼ cup almond milk

Prep time: 5 minutes

Method

- Scoop avocado flesh into a food processor or blender to prepare.
- Add almond milk, maple syrup, and chocolate powder.
- Until smooth, blend.
- Let the food cool for at least an hour in the refrigerator, before serving.

Peanut Butter and Banana Bites

Ingredients:

1 banana, cut into rounds.

1 cup of peanut butter

1 tablespoon shredded unsweetened coconut

Prep time: 5 minutes

Method

- Spread peanut butter on one side of each banana round during preparation.
- Add some coconut shreds on top.
- Offer chilled.

Veggie and Hummus Wrap

Ingredients:

1 whole wheat tortilla

2 tablespoons of hummus

1/4 cup of mixed vegetables, such as cucumber, bell peppers, and carrots

Prep time: 5 minutes

Method

- Spread hummus on the whole wheat tortilla to prepare it.
- Put hummus on top of mixed vegetables.
- The tortilla should be firmly rolled and then sliced into bite-sized pieces.

Edamame

Ingredients:

1 cup frozen edamame

Salt as desired

Prep time: 5 minutes

Method

- Prepare by bringing a kettle of water to a boil.

- Boil for 5-7 minutes after adding the frozen edamame.

- Drain and salt liberally.

Tuna and Cucumber Bites

Ingredients:

1 can drain tuna

Greek yogurt, 1/4 cup

1-tablespoon Dijon mustard

1/2 teaspoon of garlic powder

Pepper and salt as desired

Round slices of 1 cucumber

Prep time: 10 minutes

Method

- Prepare by combining the following ingredients in a bowl: tuna, Greek yogurt, Dijon mustard, garlic powder, salt, and pepper.

- On each ring of cucumber, spread the tuna mixture.
- Offer chilled.

Veggie and Cream Cheese Pinwheels

Ingredients:

1 tortilla whole-wheat

2/batch of cream cheese

1/4 cup of mixed vegetables, such as cucumber, bell peppers, and carrots

Prep time: 5 minutes

Method

- Spread cream cheese on the whole wheat tortilla to prepare it.
- The cream cheese, and then add the mixed vegetables.
- The tortilla should be firmly rolled and then sliced into bite-sized pieces.

Skewers of Grilled Cheese and Tomatoes

Ingredients:

1 piece of whole-grain bread, sliced into tiny squares

1 piece of tiny squares-cut cheddar cheese

A lone cherry tomato

One skewer

Prep time: 5 minutes

Time to cook: 5-7 minutes

Method

- Bread, cheese, and tomato are threaded onto a skewer as the preparation method.
- A grill pan should be heated to medium.
- Put the skewer on the grill pan and cook it for 5 to 7 minutes, turning it over once or twice, until the bread is toasted and the cheese has melted.

Made-at-home Trail Mix

Ingredients:

Almonds, one-fourth cup

Cashews, ¼ cup

30 grams of pumpkin seeds

¼ cup dried cranberries without added sugar

Prep time: 5 minutes

Method

- All ingredients should be combined in a bowl
- Use an airtight container for storage.

Almonds with Cinnamon Roasting

Ingredients:

Almonds, 1 cup

1-tablespoon coconut oil

1 tablespoon of honey

1 teaspoon of cinnamon

Prep time: 5 minutes

Method

- Set the oven's temperature to 350°F (180°C).
- In a basin that is microwave-safe, liquefy coconut oil.
- The heated coconut oil will be combined with honey and cinnamon after being added, add the almonds into the mixture.
- Bake for a few minutes
- Serve

Desserts and Treats with Low Sugar

Strawberry Banana Frozen Yogurt

Ingredients:

2 ripe bananas, frozen in slices.

1 cup of strawberries, frozen

Greek yogurt, plain, in 1/2 cup

1 tablespoon of honey

Prep time: 5 minutes

Method

- Greek yogurt, honey, frozen strawberries, and banana slices, all of which have to be prepared in a blender or food processor.
- Blend till creamy and smooth.
- Serve right away.

Baked Cinnamon Apple Chips

Ingredients:

2 thinly cut apples

1-tablespoon coconut oil

1 teaspoon of cinnamon

Prep time: 10 minutes

Method

- The oven should be preheated at 200°F (95°C).

- Combine cinnamon and warmed coconut oil with apple slices.
- On a baking sheet, arrange apple slices in a single layer.
- Bake until crispy in the preheated oven for 2 to 3 hours.
- Use an airtight container for storage after allowing it to cool.

Peanut Butter and Banana Bites

Ingredients:

1 banana, cut into rounds.

Natural peanut butter, 2 tablespoons

2 tablespoons shredded unsweetened coconut

Prep time: 5 minutes

Method

- Each banana circle was prepared by spreading peanut butter on it.
- Add some coconut flakes to the peanut butter.

- Offer chilled.

Berry and Greek Yogurt Parfait

Ingredients:

1 cup of Greek yogurt, plain

A half-cup of mixed berries

1/4 cup of cereal

Prep time: 5 minutes

Method

- Greek yogurt, mixed berries, and granola are layered in a glass or bowl as the preparation method.
- Continue until every ingredient has been utilized.
- Offer chilled.

Strawberries Dipped in Chocolate

Ingredients:

1 cup strawberries, please

½ cup chips of dark chocolate

Prep time: 10 minutes

Method

- Melt chocolate chips in a dish that can go in the microwave.
- The melted chocolate should be used to dip each strawberry.
- Place there to solidify on a baking sheet fitted with paper.
- Leave to chill for at least 30 minutes, then serve.

Chia Seed Dessert

Ingredients:

1 cup of almond milk without sugar

Chia seeds, 1/4 cup

1 tablespoon of honey

Vanilla extract, 1 teaspoon

Prep time: 5 minutes

Method

- Prepare by combining almond milk, chia seeds, honey, and vanilla essence in a dish.
- At least 30 minutes, or until the mixture has thickened, should be spent chilling in the refrigerator.
- Offer chilled.

Bake-Free Energy Balls

Ingredients:

1/2 cup natural peanut butter

1 cup of rolled oats.

Honey, 1/4 cup

1/4 cup coconut shreds without sugar

Prep time: 10 minutes

Method

- Prepare by combining rolled oats, peanut butter, honey, and shredded coconut in a bowl.

Create bite-sized balls of the mixture.

- Let the food cool for at least 30 minutes in the refrigerator, before you serve it.

Frozen Yogurt Bark

Ingredients:

2 cups of plain Greek yogurt

Honey and mixed berries totaling 1/4 cup

1/4 cup of cereal

Prep time: 5 minutes

Method

- Greek yogurt and honey are mixed in a bowl as the preparation method.
- On a baking sheet lined with paper, spread the mixture.
- Top the yogurt mixture with granola and a sprinkle of mixed berries.
- For at least one hour, freeze.
- Serve after breaking into pieces.

Mango Sorbet

Ingredients:

Two ripe mangos, peeled and diced.

Honey, 1/4 cup

10 ml of lime juice

Prep time: 10 minutes

Method

- Mango chunks, honey, and lime juice should be combined in a blender or food processor before serving.
- Blend till creamy and smooth.
- The mixture should be poured into a shallow dish and frozen for three hours minimum.
- To give the frozen mixture a sorbet-like texture, scrape it with a fork.
- Serve right away.

Date and Almond Butter Bars

Ingredients:

1 cup dates with pits

1/2 cup uncooked almonds

A quarter cup of almond butter

1/4 cup coconut shreds without sugar

Prep time: 10 minutes

Method

- Shredded coconut, dates, almonds, and almond butter should all be added to a food processor.
- Pulse the contents until a sticky dough forms.
- Refrigerate for at least one hour after pressing the mixture into a baking dish.
- Slice into bars, then serve.

Banana Oat Cookies

Ingredients:

2 ripe bananas, mashed

Rolled oats, 1 cup

One-fourth cup of organic peanut butter

Vanilla extract, 1 teaspoon

Prep time: 10 minutes

Method

- The oven should be preheated at 350°F (175°C).
- Bananas, rolled oats, peanut butter, and vanilla essence should all be combined in a bowl.
- Spoonfuls of the mixture should be dropped onto a parchment paper-lined baking sheet.
- Let it bake for about 10-15 minutes or until golden brown around the edges.
- After cooling, serve.

Carrot Cake Bites

Ingredients:

1 cup of grated carrots

Oats, rolled, in a cup

1/4 cup coconut shreds without sugar

1 cup of raisins

Honey, 1/4 cup

1 teaspoon of cinnamon

Prep time: 10 minutes

Method

- Shredded carrots, rolled oats, shredded coconut, raisins, honey, and cinnamon are combined in a food processor and pulsed until the ingredients form a sticky dough.
- Create bite-sized balls of the mixture.
- Let the food cool for at least 30 minutes in the refrigerator, before serving.

Lemon Blueberry Bars

Ingredients:

Almond flour, 1 cup

Melted 1/4 cup coconut oil

Honey, 1/4 cup

Fresh blueberries, half a cup

1 tablespoon each of lemon juice and zest

Prep time: 10 minutes

Method

- Set the oven's temperature to 350°F (175°C).
- Almond flour melted coconut oil, and honey should all be combined in a bowl.
- Pour the mixture into a baking pan with parchment paper-lined.
- For ten minutes, bake.
- Combine blueberries, lemon juice, and lemon zest in a separate bowl.
- On the crust that has only half cooked, pour the blueberry mixture.
- Put the dish back in the oven and bake it for 15 more minutes.
- Cut into bars after letting cool.

Chia Pudding

Ingredients:

Chia seeds, 1/4 cup

1 cup of almond milk without sugar

1 tablespoon of honey

Vanilla extract, 1 teaspoon

Prep time: 5 minutes

Method

- Chia seeds, almond milk, honey, and vanilla essence should all be combined in a bowl.

- Stir well and let aside for at least 30 minutes while stirring now and again.

- Transfer the mixture to a dish or jar after it has thickened, then serve.

- If desired, garnish with nuts or fresh fruit.

Chapter Seven

Conclusion and Future Outlook

A sugar detox diet for children has several lasting advantages. Children may enhance their energy levels, maintain a healthy weight, and improve their physical and mental health by consuming less sugar. It may be difficult for both parents and children to commit to a low-sugar diet, which is necessary to reap these advantages.

It's crucial to include kids in the process and provide them with information and tools if you want them to maintain a low-sugar lifestyle. By teaching them how to read food labels, providing healthy snacks and meals, and promoting educated decision-making, parents can empower their kids. Setting attainable objectives and acknowledging accomplishments may also keep youngsters interested and motivated.

A sugar detox diet for kids must have the support of the family to be successful. In addition to setting an example of good eating habits, parents and other caregivers are crucial in creating a nurturing atmosphere. Children are more likely to adopt and maintain a low-sugar diet when families work together to make good decisions.

Questions concerning kid-friendly sugar detox diets are also frequent. Common worries include whether it is healthy for kids to fully cut off sugar, how to handle social settings involving sugary foods, and what kinds of substitute sweeteners are kid-friendly. Families may get the answers to their concerns and make knowledgeable choices about their children's health by engaging with a trained healthcare provider and utilizing trustworthy resources.

Children's physical and mental health may greatly and long-lastingly benefit from a sugar detox diet. Parents may contribute to their children's future health and happiness by promoting a low-sugar lifestyle, offering information and tools, and cooperating as a family.